A DIY Guide for All Things Natural Hair

Discover Homemade Conditioner and Hair Rinse Recipes for Your Crowning Glory

By B. CliShea

A DIY GUIDE FOR ALL THINGS NATURAL HAIR

Discover Homemade Conditioner and Hair Rinse
Recipes for Your Crowning Glory.
By B. **CliShea**

First Edition

https://www.clishea.co/

Cover & Interior layout design by Mariana Vidakovics De Victor
Images from: https://pixabay.com/

Welcome and thank you!

This book contains awesome hair care recipes made using nutrient-rich formulas. These concoctions will help you achieve healthy, youthful, silky smooth hair!

Many commercial hair products contain harmful chemicals that may damage your hair. These chemicals seep into the scalp and can negatively affect the structure and texture of hair – thinning and weakening entire strands. These chemicals can even cause dizziness and nausea.

Well, by reading this book, you'll learn how to create all-natural treatments at home – using ingredients that you can find in your kitchen pantry. Rest assured that everything in this book is natural and simple.

To be a bit more specific, here you'll find recipes for natural leave-in conditioners, rinse-out hair conditioners, deep conditioners, and complimentary hair treatments.

By the way, because of your purchase, we are giving you a free gift. Visit my website[1] and enter your email address. We have a lot in store for you!

THANK YOU AGAIN FOR PURCHASING THIS BOOK!

---

1 https://www.instafreebie.com/free/xNCiP

Contents

Introduction 7
Commonly Known Hair Conditioners 9
  Instant/Rinse Out conditioners.......................... 10
  Leave In Conditioners 10
  Deep Conditioners 11
Complimentary Hair Treatments........................... 13
  Acid Rinses.. 13
  Herbal Rinses 15
  Beer and Alcohol Rinses 16
  Oil Conditioners 17
  Essential Oils + Carrier Oils 19
DIY Hair Conditioner Recipes 21
  Deep Conditioners 22
  Oil Conditioners 30
  Herbal Rinse 34
  Acid Rinse... 40
  Beer Rinses 45
  Instant/Rinse-out Conditioners 49
  Leave In Conditioner 55
Hair Conditioning Treatment 61
  Summary and Recommendations 61
  Benefits of Ingredients Found in Recipes 63
    Apple Cider Vinegar 63
    Aloe Vera 63
    Avocado 64
    Baking Soda 64
    Banana... 64
    Beer... 64
    Black Tea 65
    Burdock Root... 65
    Cayenne Pepper 65
    Chamomile Tea 65

Cocoa Powder 66
Coca-Cola 66
Coconut Milk 66
Coconut oil 66
Cedarwood Oil 67
Clary Sage Oil 67
Comfrey Root 67
Eggs 67
Extra Virgin Coconut Oil 67
Geranium Oil 68
Grapeseed Oil 68
Green Tea 68
Honey 68
Horsetail 68
Jojoba Oil 69
Juniper Berry Oil 69
Lavender Oil 69
Lemon 69
Lemon Grass Essential Oil 70
Mayonnaise 70
Nettle 70
Olive Oil 70
Peppermint Oil and Leaves 70
Rooibois Tea 71
Raspberry Leaves 71
Rose Essential Oil 71
Rosehip Oil 71
Rosemary Essential Oil 72
Sandalwood Oil 72
Shea butter 72
Strawberry 72
Sweet Almond Oil 72
Tea Tree Oil 73
Thyme 73
Vanilla Essential Oil 73

Vegetable Glycerin 73
Virgin Coconut Oil 73
Witch Hazel.. 74
Ylang ylang Oil.. 74
Yogurt 74
Conclusion... 75
Resources.. 77

Introduction

Your hair is your crowning glory, so you have to nourish it with all-natural products. But, why should you spend your precious time making homemade rinses and conditioners when you can purchase hair care products at the grocery store?

Generally, hair care products are designed to strengthen the hair follicles, revitalize the scalp, and nourish the roots. They help seal hair color, repair damage, prevent split ends, and give hair a soft and silky finish.

Well, this may be a bitter pill to swallow, but a lot of hair care products on the market today contain chemicals that may damage your hair and even your health. Synthetic hair care products contain ingredients that are also used in other products such as plastics, motor lubricants, refrigerants, insect repellants, fuel gas, paint, and furniture finishers. These ingredients are absorbed into your scalp and then, they are transported in your bloodstream. The toxins contained in these ingredients can cause hair and skin dryness, hair thinning, and hair loss. But, they can also cause more serious problems like allergic reactions, eczema, skin damage, eye irritation, lung damage, kidney damage, and asphyxiation.

To avoid health problems and other complications, it's good to use natural homemade products.

Using homemade hair care products has a lot of benefits, including:

* Homemade hair care products contain ingredients that are rich in vitamins and minerals, making your hair healthier and more beautiful.
* Over-the-counter organic hair care products cost a lot of money. So, making hair care products at home can help you save.
* Homemade hair care products do not contain harmful ingredients such as ammonium lauryl sulfate, sodium lauryl sulfate, propylene glycol, myreth sulfate, and olefin sulfonate.
* When you use hair care products that contain toxic chemicals, you are poisoning your body. So, using all-natural homemade hair care products reduces your toxin intake and improves your overall health.
* A lot of homemade hair care products yield instant results.
* They are easy to make. It usually takes less than ten minutes to make a homemade hair conditioner.
* You do not have to spend hundreds of dollars to make your hair shinier and more beautiful. All you need to do is whip up a few food items that you can find in your kitchen!

Commonly Known Hair Conditioners

Shampoo is good for your hair. It cleanses your hair and removes dirt. It also reduces the itchiness, inflammation, and redness of the scalp. It controls the oiliness of your hair and it keeps the hair beautiful. Some shampoos also remove dandruff.

But, shampooing every day can potentially damage your hair, particularly the follicles. Frequent shampooing depletes the moisture and nutrition of your hair. This is the reason why it's important to use a conditioner.

A good conditioner moisturizes your scalp and restores the natural luster of your hair. It prevents hair damage and fights dryness. Conditioners provide immediate benefits. This means you get shinier hair right away.

Keep in mind though, that not all hair conditioners are the same. To help you learn about their differences, here's a list of commonly known hair conditioners:

Instant/Rinse Out conditioners

Instant conditioners coat hair well. They temporarily soothe your hair, making it shiny and easy to style. You should apply an instant conditioner right after you rinse out your shampoo. You should leave it on for two to three minutes. Be sure to completely rinse it off afterwards.

This is great for detangling the hair, but it has a thinner consistency. This type of conditioner is perfect for hair that's minimally damaged as it does not repair extreme hair damage. Rinse-out conditioners are usually cheaper and easier to find.

Instant conditioners protect the hair from thermal damage and lock out humidity. These make combing easier and are easy to use.

Rinse-out conditioners are naturally heavier and thicker than most leave-in treatments. That's because the former coat the hair strand with a thick layer that tightly sticks to hair even after rinsing.

You should apply this conditioner right after you shampoo, once every two days.

Leave In Conditioners

Leave-in conditioners enhance the softness of hair. They also retain both moisture and shine. You need to apply this kind of conditioner after you rinse out your shampoo. But, you do not have to rinse it out. You can leave it on your hair as you go about your day.

A leave-in conditioner will nourish your hair, giving it a silky and luminous glow. It can be used between washes and it makes your hair more manageable.

This type of conditioner comes in different forms (liquid, sprays, or thick creams) so its consistency and texture varies. Still, leave-in conditioners are generally watery and much lighter compared to rinse-out conditioners.

A leave-in conditioner is a powerful moisturizer that can tame frizzy hair. So, it's best for kinkier and curly hair types. It loosens the waves, making hair shiny and soft. It detangles knotted hair and helps prevent breakage. It smoothens the split ends and protects hair from environmental damage. It also adds luster and gloss to color-treated hair. It coats the outer layer of hair, adding smoothness and softness.

There's a number of good quality leave-in conditioners on the market today, such as the Aphogee Keratin and Green Restructurizer, Luster's S-Curl No Drip Activator Moisturizer, Elasta QP Feels Like Silk Leave-in Conditioning Repair Cream, and Herbal Essences Beautiful Ends.

To use a leave-in conditioner, dry your hair using a towel after rinsing out the shampoo. Then, apply the conditioner from root to tip. But, focus on the ends as they are the weakest part of your hair. Do not apply too much conditioner as this could weigh down your hair.

Deep Conditioners

Deep conditioners improve the look and health of hair. However, you need to apply heat treatment for these conditioners to work. You should apply a deep conditioner after washing your hair, leaving it on for twenty to thirty minutes. You also need to apply heat treatment (you can use a warm wet towel or a hair dryer).

Deep conditioners are great hair moisturizers, enhancing your hair's shine and luster. They soften hair and even repair dry and damaged hair. They also reduce frizz.

Deep conditioners are powerful enough to prevent damage and improve moisture. They promote elasticity and enhance both luster and shine. These conditioners contain essential natural oils, water, and protein – all of which moisturize your hair.

This type of conditioner is best for people with dry and damaged hair. It also improves the shine of color-treated hair.

Shampoo can do wonders to your hair, but it's not enough. You need to condition your hair, too.

Complimentary Hair Treatments

Applying chemicals to your hair can lead to damage in the long run. Rinses are complimentary treatments that restore balance, healing damaged hair naturally. Aside from that, they improve the blood circulation in your scalp, leading to faster hair growth.

What's amazing about hair rinses is that they are made of natural ingredients that you can find in your kitchen. They are both effective and inexpensive.

Acid Rinses

Acid rinses smoothens the hair from the shaft down to the tip. They help remove tangles and counteract the harmful effects of alkaline shampoo.

1. Apple Cider Vinegar

Apple cider vinegar is a natural hair conditioner that improves the shine of your hair. It has both short- and long-term effects. For best results, use apple cider three times a week.

2. Lemon Juice

Drinking lemon juice can do wonders to your digestive system and your skin. But, do you know that lemon juice is good for your hair, too? It can treat a wide array of hair problems including hair loss and dandruff. Lemon juice enhances the luster and shine of your hair. It also creates beautiful and natural highlights.

Lemon juice has strong astringent qualities that can tighten your pores and skin. When the pores in your scalp shrink, the oil doesn't seep out. So, lemon rinse is best for those who have oily hair.

Do a lemon rinse for five minutes to lighten hair and to tighten the scalp's pores. Lemon juice is strong though, meaning you should only apply it once every two weeks.

3. Coca-Cola

Yes, you've read it right. If this hair rinse is good enough for Suki Waterhouse, it's definitely good enough for us. Coke may not be the healthiest drink, but it can do wonders to your hair. It increases volume and makes curls bigger and more defined. Simply put, if you want to achieve Beyonce's sassy curls, it's a good idea to rinse your hair with this fizzy drink.

If you have short hair, you can simply use one 350 ml can of Coke. But, if you have long hair, you'll be needing two cans.

A Coca-Cola rinse works best on thin and limp hair. To rinse your hair with Coke, pour a can or two in a huge bowl or small basin. Then, dip your head into the bowl and make sure that your hair is deeply coated. Leave it on for one to two minutes. Then, rinse it thoroughly with water.

Dry your hair using a blower afterwards. When your hair is completely dry, you'll notice that it has more volume.

This rinse is cheap and it makes your hair soft. It creates beautiful and natural waves, too! Remember not to overdo it though. Once a month or once every two months should be enough.

Herbal Rinses

Herbal rinses are packed with nutrients and antioxidants. These rinses invigorate your scalp and hair.

1. Peppermint Tea

Peppermint tea is powerful yet easy to use. Just pour the rinse over your hair and leave it on for 30 minutes. Put on a shower cap. After a few minutes, rinse your hair with cold water. Apply this rinse once a week.

2. Black Tea

Black tea decreases the level of dihydrotestosterone – a hormone that causes baldness. This hair rinse increases hair thickness and stimulates hair growth. It improves shine as well. It even darkens hair, making it perfect for those with graying manes. To use black tea, just leave it on your hair for an hour. After that, rinse it thoroughly. You may enjoy this rinse once a week.

3. Roboois Tea

Roboois tea is filled with antioxidants. It improves hair growth since its rich in nutrients such as potassium, copper, calcium, and zinc. It has a strengthening effect so it's quite perfect for color-treated hair. Leave it on your hair for 30 to 40 minutes, then rinse. Apply it twice a week for best results.

4. Green Tea

Green tea balances the pH levels of your scalp. It also normalizes oil production and controls dandruff. Green tea contains vitamin C, vitamin E, and polyphenols that protect hair from sun damage. This rinse can repair hair damage and prevents split ends, too. Pour the rinse over dry or damp hair and leave it on for 30 to 40 minutes. Use it at least once a week.

Beer and Alcohol Rinses

Beer is good for your hair. It repairs hair damage and improves volume.

1. Beer Rinse

Who would have thought that beer is the key to having beautiful and lustrous hair? It makes your hair shiny and adds volume. It also strengthens your hair and is a known solution to oiliness in the scalp. To use beer as a rinse, simply pour it over your hair. Leave it on for 30 minutes before rinsing off with cold water.

2. Champagne

Champagne is expensive. But, if you have money to burn, you can use champagne as a hair rinse. It is rich in antioxidants (Vitamins C and E) that make hair glossier and shinier.

Pour the champagne over your damp hair and leave it on for 45 minutes before rinsing. Use once a month, but don't hesitate to try other rinses if this one doesn't provide noticeable results right away.

Oil Conditioners

Oil conditioners have an instant effect. They are perfect for dull and dry hair.

1. Coconut Oil

Coconut oil fights infection with its strong anti-fungal properties. It's also a good styling agent, being capable of fighting even the worst frizz.

Massage coconut oil into your hair. Do not apply too much on your scalp as this may clog the pores. Apply this at least once every two weeks.

2. Olive Oil

Olive oil is a powerful conditioner that increases luster. It smoothens hair and helps prevent split ends. It even reduces dandruff and helps eliminate head lice.

Apply olive oil on your hair after rinsing off the shampoo. Leave it on for 30 to 40 minutes, then rinse it off. You can use this conditioner once or twice a week.

3. Almond Oil

This oil is packed with nutrients such as vitamin E, magnesium, and omega-3 fatty acids. It penetrates your hair easily, so you'll see instant results. It smells good, too. Keep in mind though, that almond oil is best for dry and brittle hair.

To use almond oil, just apply it on your hair. Massage it from the root of your hair to the tip. Leave it on for 30 minutes and rinse off with cold water. Use it once a week.

4. Jojoba Oil

This oil is a popular shampoo ingredient. It moisturizes hair, helps reduce dandruff, and cuts scalp dryness. This wonder oil contains vitamin B, vitamin E, zinc, copper, silicon, and copper.

Apply to your hair after shower. Place a warm towel over your head and leave it on for 30 minutes. Then, rinse it off. This moisturizer produces quick results, but you also need to use it regularly to see long-term results. Use it twice a week for at least eight weeks.

Essential Oils + Carrier Oils

Essential oils can do wonders to your health – and they can make your hair more beautiful, too. Essential oils are strong so you just need to mix a few drops of each mixed with a cup of carrier oil such as sweet almond oil, olive oil, and jojoba oil.

1. Chamomile Oil + Olive Oil

Chamomile is rich in antioxidants and strengthens hair.

* Best for brittle and stressed hair
* Add five drops of chamomile oil to one cup of olive oil
* Apply on damp hair after rinsing off the shampoo.
* Leave it on for 10 to 20 minutes. Then, rinse of the oil thoroughly.

2. Clary Sage Oil + Jojoba Oil

Clary sage oil regulates the production of oil in the scalp. It contains a strong anti-bacterial agent, relieves stress, and prevents hair loss.

* Great for oily hair
* Controls dandruff
* Reinvigorates hair
* Combine one cup of jojoba oil and five drops of clary sage oil. Massage it into the scalp and leave it on for 30 minutes. Afterwards, rinse it off with cold water.

3. Lavender Oil + Olive Oil

Lavender oil has strong antimicrobial properties.

It promotes hair growth and it's best for thinning and balding hair.

* It soothes the scalp and heals dry skin
* Mix 2 tablespoons of olive oil, ½ cup of water, and ten drops of lavender oil. Massage into your hair. Leave it on for 30 minutes. Rinse it off.
  Use this conditioner once every two weeks.

4. Rosemary Oil + Sweet Almond Oil

Rosemary oil increases the thickness of hair. It promotes hair growth and prevents baldness. It also slows down the graying process. It treats dandruff, too.

* Combine ½ cup of almond oil and ten drops of rosemary oil
* Massage the conditioner into your scalp. Leave it on for 30 minutes and then rinse it off.

5. Lemongrass Essential Oil + Jojoba Oil

Lemongrass strengthens hair, while helping ease scalp irritation. It also reduces hair stress and gives hair a bit more shine. To prepare this concoction, combine ½ cup of jojoba oil with 10 drops of lemongrass essential oil. Apply the conditioner to your hair. Wrap your hair in a warm towel. Leave it on for 30 minutes. Rinse off the oil using cold water.

Complimentary hair treatments help you achieve glossier and shinier hair. These treatments are not as harsh as color or chemical treatments. They also help repair sun damage, making your hair healthier and more beautiful.

DIY Hair Conditioner Recipes

DIY hair conditioners are incredibly easy to make. In fact, it takes less than ten minutes to make most of the hair conditioner recipes listed in this book.

Here's are the tools that you'll need:

1. Mixing bowls
2. Plastic containers
3. Water bottles
4. Small dark glass bottles
5. Cheese cloth and string
6. Herbs and teas
7. Fresh food items
8. Cooking pot
9. Metal containers

You can find the containers at a local beauty shop. Of course, you can also get them online.

You'll find essential oils in beauty shops and on the web. Make sure to go for "pure essential oils" and not the "fragrance" variety.

As for the herbs, you can get most of them in Chinese, Korean, or Japanese herbal stores. You can also plant some of these herbs in your backyard.

Deep Conditioners

Recipe #1

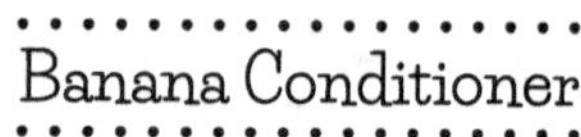

Banana Conditioner

INGREDIENT LIST
- 4 tablespoons of extra virgin coconut oil
- 2 tablespoons of honey
- 2 tablespoons of vegetable glycerin
- 1 large banana (you can also use banana baby food)

STEP-BY-STEP INSTRUCTIONS
1. Slice the banana and place it in a blender.
2. Add the glycerin, honey, and virgin coconut oil.
3. Process for 30 seconds to one minute.
4. Transfer the conditioner into a bowl.

HAIR APPLICATION DIRECTIONS

Apply the banana conditioner on dry hair, massaging gently. Cover your hair with a warm towel and let the conditioner sit for 30 minutes. Then, rinse your hair with cold water.

STORAGE OF PRODUCT

It's best to use this conditioner right away. But, if you want to store this, you can place it in a plastic container. Be sure to keep it in the fridge.

SHELF LIFE

This conditioner only lasts for about 48 hours.

Recipe #2

Shea Butter and Avocado

Ingredient List

- ¼ cup of extra virgin coconut oil
- 1 avocado
- 3 tablespoons of apple cider vinegar
- ½ cup of shea butter

Step-by-step Instructions

1. Place the apple cider vinegar, shea butter, avocado, and extra virgin coconut oil. You do not have to melt the shea butter ahead.

2. Process for one minute.

3. Transfer the mixture in a bowl.

Hair Application Directions

Shampoo your hair. After rinsing out the shampoo, apply the conditioner. Cover with a warm towel. You can also place a shower cap over your hair and then, place a blower near the shower cap for about one minute. Let the conditioner sit for 30 to 45 minutes. This conditioner is a natural detangler.

Storage of Product

Place the remaining conditioner in a small plastic container and store in the refrigerator.

Shelf Life

It is best to use this product right after mixing it. However, you can store it in the refrigerator up to 48 hours.

<u>**Recipe #3**</u>

Classic Egg Yolk Conditioner

INGREDIENT LIST
- 1 egg yolk
- 2 tablespoons of olive oil
- 2 spoons of mayonnaise

STEP-BY-STEP INSTRUCTIONS
1. Place the egg yolk, olive oil, and mayonnaise in a bowl.
2. Mix all the ingredients using a fork.

HAIR APPLICATION DIRECTIONS
Apply the conditioner on dry hair. Blow dry your hair for you about one minute. Leave the conditioner on for 30 to 40 minutes. Rinse off using lukewarm water.

STORAGE OF PRODUCT
You can store the product in a small plastic or glass container. Then, store it in the refrigerator.

SHELF LIFE
This conditioner can last up to five days.

<u>Recipe #4</u>

DIY Coconut Oil Conditioner

INGREDIENT LIST
- 3 spoons of coconut milk
- 2 spoons of olive oil
- 2 drops rosemary oil

STEP-BY-STEP INSTRUCTIONS
1. Combine the ingredients in a small bowl.
2. Stir well and let it set for a few minutes before using.

HAIR APPLICATION DIRECTIONS
Massage the hair conditioner on your hair (make sure your hair is covered from root to tip).

STORAGE OF PRODUCT
Store the conditioner in a cool, dark place. You can also refrigerate it to extend its shelf life.

SHELF LIFE
This hair conditioner lasts for one week when stored properly. But, if you refrigerate it, it can last for up to two months (rosemary oil is a natural preservative).

Recipe #5

DIY Yogurt Hair Conditioner

INGREDIENT LIST

- 2 cups of yogurt
- 2 tablespoons of virgin coconut oil
- 2 tablespoons of castor oil

STEP-BY-STEP INSTRUCTIONS

1. Whip the yogurt in a bowl.
2. Stir in the castor oil and the virgin coconut oil.
3. Mix the ingredients well.

HAIR APPLICATION DIRECTIONS

Apply this conditioner on dry hair. Massage your hair well. Wrap your hair with a warm towel. Leave it on for 30 to 40 minutes.

STORAGE OF PRODUCT

Just transfer the conditioner in a plastic container and refrigerate immediately.

SHELF LIFE

This concoction lasts up to a week.

Recipe #6

Yogurt and Aloe Vera Conditioner

Ingredient List
- 3 drops of tea tree oil
- 1 cup of plain Greek yogurt
- 2 tablespoons of aloe vera gel
- 1 tablespoon of olive oil

Step-by-step Instructions
1. Place all the ingredients in a bowl.
2. Mix well.

Hair Application Directions
Apply the conditioner on damp hair. Cover your hair with a plastic conditioning cap. Leave the conditioner on for one hour. Apply this at least once a week.

Storage of Product
Place the mixture in a small plastic container. Store in the refrigerator.

Shelf Life
This hair conditioner lasts up to 72 hours.

Recipe #7

Egg and Olive Oil Mask

INGREDIENT LIST
- 2 teaspoons of olive oil
- 2 tablespoons of jojoba oil
- ½ cup of water
- 2 egg yolks

STEP-BY-STEP INSTRUCTIONS
1. Place the egg yolk in a bowl. Stir.
2. Add the olive oil and jojoba oil.
3. Add the water.
4. Stir well.

HAIR APPLICATION DIRECTIONS
Massage the mixture onto damp hair. Place a conditioning cap on your hair. Leave it on for 45 minutes. Remove the cap and rinse off the conditioner thoroughly.

STORAGE OF PRODUCT
Place the conditioner in a plastic container. Then, store in the refrigerator.

SHELF LIFE
This conditioner stays good for two to three days.

Recipe #8

Vinegar and Mayonnaise Invigorating Conditioner

INGREDIENT LIST

- ½ cup of mayonnaise
- ¼ cup of apple cider vinegar
- ½ cup of jojoba oil

STEP-BY-STEP INSTRUCTIONS

1. Place the mayonnaise, jojoba oil, and apple cider vinegar in a small bowl.

2. Mix well.

HAIR APPLICATION DIRECTIONS

Apply the conditioner on dry hair. Massage into your hair from the root to the tip. Now, blow dry your hair for about one minute. Place a shower cap on your hair and leave it on for 30 to 45 minutes. Remove the shower cap and rinse off the conditioner.

STORAGE OF PRODUCT

Place this conditioner in a bowl or a plastic container and then place in the refrigerator.

SHELF LIFE

This conditioner lasts three to seven days.

Oil Conditioners

Recipe #9

Lavender and Chocolate Conditioner

INGREDIENT LIST

- 2 cups of Greek yogurt
- 10 drops of rose hip seed oil
- 6 drops of lavender oil
- ½ cup of raw Cacao powder
- 3 tablespoons of coconut oil
- 1 cup of sweet almond oil

STEP-BY-STEP INSTRUCTIONS

1. Whip the Greek yogurt in a bowl.
2. Add the cocoa powder and stir well.
3. Add the rose hip seed oil, coconut oil, and lavender oil.
4. Stir well.

HAIR APPLICATION DIRECTIONS

Apply the conditioner on damp hair. Put on a conditioning cap and allow the conditioner to sit for 45 minutes.

STORAGE OF PRODUCT

Place the conditioner in a plastic container. Then, store in the refrigerator.

SHELF LIFE

This conditioner stays good for three to five days.

Recipe #10

Hair Growth Rinse

INGREDIENT LIST
- 1 cup of extra virgin coconut oil
- 10 drops of rosemary oil
- 5 drops of cedarwood essential oil

STEP-BY-STEP INSTRUCTIONS
1. Combine all the ingredients in a bowl.
2. Stir for about 30 seconds to make sure that the ingredients are mixed well.

HAIR APPLICATION DIRECTIONS
Apply the conditioner on damp hair. Massage your hair thoroughly, allowing the nutrients to seep in. Leave the conditioner on for 30 minutes. Then, rinse off using cold water.

STORAGE OF PRODUCT
For maximum shelf life, refrigerate the conditioner. However, it's perfectly fine to simply store it in a cool and dark place.

SHELF LIFE
The regular shelf life of this conditioner is three months. But, it can last up to six months if kept in the fridge.

<u>Recipe #11</u>

Clary Sage, Aloe Vera, and Tea Tree Oil Mix

INGREDIENT LIST

- 10 drops of clary sage essential oil
- 10 drops of aloe vera oil
- 10 drops of tea tree oil
- 2 drops of rosemary oil
- 1 cup of jojoba oil

STEP-BY-STEP INSTRUCTIONS

1. Place the water in a medium-sized bowl.

2. Add ten drops of clary sage essential oil. Then, stir the mixture.

3. Add ten drops of aloe vera oil and stir well.

4. Add ten drops of tea tree oil.

5. Stir well.

HAIR APPLICATION DIRECTIONS

Apply this conditioner on damp hair. Place a shower cap and leave the conditioner on for 30 to 45 minutes.

STORAGE OF PRODUCT

Place the remaining conditioner in a small plastic bottle. You can also place it in a spray bottle. Store this conditioner in a cool, dark place.

SHELF LIFE

This mixture can last up to six months.

Recipe #12

Juniper Berry Oil Rinse

INGREDIENT LIST
- 1 cup of sweet almond oil
- 15 drops of juniper berry oil
- 2 drops of rosemary oil
- 1/4 cup of fresh crushed aloe vera gel

STEP-BY-STEP INSTRUCTIONS
1. Place the water and the aloe vera gel in the blender.
2. Process for 30 seconds.
3. Transfer the mixture into a plastic bottle.
4. Add the juniper oil and rosemary oil.
5. Shake well. Let the mixture sit for at least one hour before using.

HAIR APPLICATION DIRECTIONS
Massage the mixture onto damp hair. Be sure to massage thoroughly for two to three minutes. Place a conditioning cap on your hair and let the mixture sit for 30 minutes.

STORAGE OF PRODUCT
Store the conditioner in a cold and dark place. You can also place it in the refrigerator.

SHELF LIFE
This conditioner lasts up to 30 days. But, it can last longer if refrigerated.

Herbal Rinse

Recipe #13

Black Tea Rinse

INGREDIENT LIST
- 5 black tea bags
- 3 tablespoons of crushed rosemary leaves
- 3 tablespoons of crushed sage leaves
- Cheesecloth
- String
- 5 cups of water

STEP-BY-STEP INSTRUCTIONS
1. Place the tea bags, crushed rosemary leaves, and sage leaves on a cheese cloth. Tie the cheesecloth using a string and set aside.
2. Heat the water in a pot.
3. Place the cheesecloth in the pot (with the herbs) and bring to boil.
4. Let the mixture simmer for about five minutes.
5. Remove the pot from heat.
6. Let the mixture cool for 15 minutes.
7. Remove the cheese cloth.
8. Then, use a cheese cloth to drain the remaining leaves, if there's any.
9. Place the mixture in a plastic or glass bottle.

Place your hair over a sink. Then, pour the rinse over your hair. Massage your hair, allowing the nutrients to seep into your hair follicles and scalp. Place a shower cap over your hair and leave it on for 30 to 45 minutes. Afterwards, rinse your hair thoroughly with cold water.

Storage of Product

It's best to keep it in the fridge for maximum shelf life.

Shelf Life

This rinse can last up to a month if properly refrigerated.

Recipe #14

Green Tea Herbal Mix

Ingredient List

- 1 teaspoon of baking soda
- 5 bags of green tea
- 1 tablespoon of ground comfrey root
- 1 tablespoon of ground burdock root
- 2 tablespoons of ground nettle leaves
- Cheesecloth
- 7 cups of water

Step-by-step Instructions

1. Place the green tea, comfrey root, burdock root, and nettle leaves on a medium-sized cheese cloth.

2. Tie the cheesecloth and set aside.

3. Heat the water in a pot.

4. Place the cheese cloth in the pot.

5. Bring the mixture to boil. The water will slowly turn green.

6. Simmer for five minutes.

7. Remove the pot from heat and let it cool for 10 to 15 minutes.

8. Drain the remaining leaves, if there's any, using a clean cheesecloth.

9. Place the mixture in a plastic water bottle. You'll probably need two 500ml water bottles.

Hair Application Directions

After rinsing off your shampoo, pour this mixture over your hair. Make sure that your hair is evenly covered.

Storage of Product

Store this rinse in a dark and cool place. Refrigerate it to increase its shelf life.

Shelf Life

This rinse lasts up to seven days, though it can last up to 30 days if refrigerated.

Recipe #15

Black Tea and Raspberry Mix

Ingredient List

- 5 black tea bags
- 5 tablespoons of crushed red raspberry leaves
- 1 tablespoon of rosemary leaves
- 1 tablespoon of sage leaves
- Cheese cloth
- 7 cups of water

1. Place the tea bags, raspberry leaves, sage leaves, and rosemary leaves on the cheesecloth.
2. Tie the cloth using a string.
3. Place the water in a pot under medium heat.
4. Add the herbs (placed in the cheesecloth).
5. Bring to a boil.
6. Simmer for five to ten minutes.
7. Let the mixture cool for a few minutes.
8. Pour the mixture into a plastic bottle.

HAIR APPLICATION DIRECTIONS

Place your hair over a sink, then pour this mixture. Massage your hair for about two minutes. Wrap your hair using a warm towel. Leave it on for 30 to 45 minutes.

STORAGE OF PRODUCT

Store this product somewhere cool and dark. You can also refrigerate it to extend its shelf life.

SHELF LIFE

This hair rinse lasts for about a week. However, it can last up to a month when refrigerated.

Recipe #16

Roobois Tea and Parsley Mix

INGREDIENT LIST
- 5 roobois tea bags
- 2 tablespoons of shredded parsley leaves
- 1 tablespoon of rosemary leaves
- Cheese cloth
- String
- 5 cups of water

STEP-BY-STEP INSTRUCTIONS
1. Place the tea bags, rosemary leaves, and parsley leaves in the cheesecloth.
2. Tie the cheesecloth using a string.
3. Place five cups of water in a pot over medium heat.
4. Place the cheesecloth in the pot.
5. Bring to a boil.
6. Simmer for five minutes.
7. Remove the pot from heat and let it cool for a few minutes.
8. Pour the rinse into a plastic water bottle.

HAIR APPLICATION DIRECTIONS

Place your dry hair over a sink and pour the rinse over your head. You can also do this after applying shampoo. Massage your hair thoroughly and make sure that your hair is well-covered.

Store the rinse in a dark, cool place. You can also refrigerate it to increase its shelf life.

Shelf Life

This rinse usually lasts up to seven days. If kept in the fridge, it will stay good for up to a month.

Recipe #17

. . . .
Green Tea Anti-Dandruff Rinse
. . . .

Ingredient List
- 1 tablespoon of ground horsetail
- 1 tablespoon of crushed peppermint leaves
- 1 tablespoon of sage leaves
- 5 bags of green tea
- 5 cups of water
- Cheesecloth

Step-by-step Instructions
1. Place the horsetail, peppermint leaves, green tea bags, and sage leaves in a cheesecloth.
2. Tie the cheesecloth using a string.
3. Place five cups of water in a pot over medium heat. Add the cheesecloth to the pot and bring to boil.
4. Then, remove the pot from the heat.
5. Let the mixture cool for about ten minutes.
6. Transfer the rinse into a water bottle.

HAIR APPLICATION DIRECTIONS

After rinsing out your shampoo, pour the rinse on your hair. Then, massage your hair thoroughly to make sure that the nutrients seep into your scalp. Place a shower cap over your head. Leave it on for 30 to 45 minutes. Then, wash your hair with lukewarm water.

STORAGE OF PRODUCT

Store the rinse in a dark and cool place. It's also a good idea to refrigerate it if you want to extend its shelf life.

SHELF LIFE

This rinse typically lasts up to a week. But, it can last up to one month if you refrigerate it.

Acid Rinse

Recipe #18

Apple Cider and Lavender Hair Rinse

INGREDIENT LIST
- 2 tablespoons of dried lavender flowers
- 1 tablespoon of witch hazel
- 1 tablespoon of ground thyme leaves
- 500 ml of apple cider vinegar
- 3 cups of water

STEP-BY-STEP INSTRUCTIONS
1. Place 3 cups of water in a pot over medium heat.

2. Add the lavender flowers, thyme leaves, and witch hazel.

3. Bring to a boil.

4. Then, add the apple cider vinegar.

5. Remove the mixture from the pot.

6. Let it cool for 10 to 15 minutes.

7. Then, transfer the mixture in a water bottle.

8. Refrigerate the mixture overnight.

HAIR APPLICATION DIRECTIONS

Place your hair over a sink. Then, pour the rinse over your head. Massage your hair from root to tip. Afterwards, place a warm towel on your hair. Leave it on for 30 minutes. Remove the towel and rinse your hair with cold water.

STORAGE OF PRODUCT

Store the product in the refrigerator.

SHELF LIFE

This rinse could last up to two weeks.

Recipe #19

Lavender Oil and Apple Cider Acid Rinse

INGREDIENT LIST

- 3 cups of apple cider vinegar
- 3 cups of water
- 10 drops of lavender essential oil
- 10 drops of lemon essential oil
- 5 drops of rosemary essential oil
- 5 drops of rose oil

Step-by-step Instructions

1. Place the water in a pot over low heat.
2. Stir in the apple cider vinegar.
3. Simmer for about three minutes.
4. Add the lavender, lemon, rose, and rosemary essential oils.
5. Remove the mixture from the heat.
6. Stir well.
7. Let the mixture cool for about 15 to 30 minutes.
8. Place the rinse in a water bottle.

Hair Application Directions

Apply the rinse on damp hair. Massage your hair thoroughly. Place a shower cap over your head and leave it on for 45 minutes. Rinse out the mixture using cold water.

Storage of Product

Store the mixture in the refrigerator.

Shelf Life

This conditioner lasts up to two weeks.

Recipe #20

Apple Cider and Cayenne Pepper Rinse

Ingredient List

- 3 cups of water
- 2 cups of apple cider vinegar
- 1 teaspoon of cayenne pepper
- 2 tablespoons of ground lavender flowers
- 2 tablespoons of rosemary leaves

Step-by-Step Instructions

1. Place the water in a pot over medium heat.
2. Add the apple cider vinegar, cayenne pepper, rosemary leaves, and lavender flowers.
3. Bring to boil.
4. Simmer for five minutes.
5. Remove the pot from the heat.
6. Let the mixture cool in for 10 to 15 minutes.
7. Drain out the leaves using a cheese cloth.
8. Transfer the hair rinse in a water bottle.

Hair Application Directions

Pour the mixture on your damp hair. Massage your hair thoroughly. Place a shower cap on your head. Then, leave it on for 30 to 45 minutes. Remove the cap and rinse your hair with lukewarm water.

Storage of Product

Store the hair rinse in the refrigerator.

Shelf Life

This rinse lasts up to two weeks.

Recipe #21

Apple Cider Vinegar and Chamomile Mix

Ingredient List

- 2 cups of water
- 3 cups of apple cider vinegar
- 1 tablespoon of rosemary leaves
- 1 tablespoon of lavender flowers
- 5 drops of chamomile essential oil

1. Place the water in a cooking pot over low heat.

2. Add the apple cider vinegar, rosemary leaves, and lavender flowers.

3. Bring the mixture to boil and simmer for five minutes.

4. Remove the pot from heat and add the chamomile oil.

5. Stir well.

6. Let the mixture cool for 15 to 30 minutes.

7. Pour the mixture into the water bottle.

Hair Application Directions

Pour the acid rinse on your hair. Massage your hair from root to tip. Then, place a shower cap on your head. Leave it on for 45 minutes. Rinse your hair thoroughly with cold water. Blow dry your hair for best results.

Storage of Product

Store this rinse in the refrigerator.

Shelf Life

This rinse can last up to two weeks.

Beer Rinses

Recipe #22

Beer and Honey

INGREDIENT LIST
- 3 egg yolks
- 1 cup of beer
- 1 banana
- ¼ cup of honey

STEP-BY-STEP INSTRUCTIONS
1. Slice the banana and place it in a bowl.
2. Mash it using a spoon.
3. Add the eggs and mix thoroughly.
4. Add the beer and the honey.
5. Stir well.

HAIR APPLICATION DIRECTIONS
Pour the mixture on damp hair and leave it on for 30 minutes. Rinse thoroughly using lukewarm water.

STORAGE OF PRODUCT
You can refrigerate the remaining conditioner.

SHELF LIFE
This mixture only lasts anywhere from 24 to 48 hours.

Recipe #23

Apple Cider Vinegar and Beer

INGREDIENT LIST
- 2 cups of apple cider vinegar
- ½ cup of beer

STEP-BY-STEP INSTRUCTIONS
1. Place the ACV and the beer in a bowl.
2. Stir well.

HAIR APPLICATION DIRECTIONS

Apply the mixture on damp hair. Massage it on your scalp and roots. Massage for around two to three minutes then rinse.

STORAGE OF PRODUCT

Store the product in a plastic container or a bottle.

SHELF LIFE

This conditioner lasts for up to two weeks.

Recipe #24

Avocado, Egg, and Beer Mix

INGREDIENT LIST

- 1 cup of flat beer
- 2 eggs
- 2 tablespoons of avocado oil

STEP-BY-STEP INSTRUCTIONS

1. Crack the eggs open and place them in a bowl.
2. Beat the eggs.
3. Stir in the beer and the avocado oil.
4. Mix well.

HAIR APPLICATION DIRECTIONS

Massage the mixture to the roots of your hair. Then, apply it to the rest of your hair. Cover your hair with a shower cap. Leave it on for 30 minutes.

STORAGE OF PRODUCT

Place the mixture in a plastic container. Then, refrigerate it.

SHELF LIFE

This conditioner stays good for 48 to 72 hours.

Recipe #25

Strawberry and Beer Mix

INGREDIENT LIST

- 1 cup of sliced ripe strawberries
- 1 cup of beer

STEP-BY-STEP INSTRUCTIONS

1. Place the strawberries and beer in a blender.
2. Process for 30 to 60 seconds.
3. Place the mixture in a bowl.

HAIR APPLICATION DIRECTIONS

Apply the mixture on dry hair. Massage it into your hair – from root to tip. Wrap your hair with a warm towel. Wait for 30 minutes. Afterwards, rinse the conditioner out with lukewarm water.

STORAGE OF PRODUCT

Place the mixture in a plastic container and then refrigerate.

SHELF LIFE

You can use this mixture within 3 to 7 days.

Instant/Rinse-out Conditioners

It is fairly easy to make a rinse-out conditioner. You can find most of the ingredients for these recipes in your kitchen. You can also buy the essential oils at your local health stores. However, if you want to purchase a pre-made conditioner base, simply visit these web pages:

* Brambleberry.com, our favorite conditioner recipe[2]
* Organic-creations.com, hair conditioner base[3]
* Brambleberry.com, stephenson organic conditioner[4]

Recipe #26

Olive Oil Homemade Instant Conditioner

INGREDIENT LIST
- 3 drops of lavender essential oil
- 3 drops of rose oil
- 1 cup of extra virgin olive oil
- 3 drops of vanilla oil

STEP-BY-STEP INSTRUCTIONS
1. Place the extra virgin olive oil in a bowl.
2. Add rose oil, lavender oil, and vanilla oil.
3. Mix well.
4. Place the mixture in a small dark bottle.

---

2 https://www.brambleberry.com/our-favorite-conditioner-recipe.aspx
3 http://www.organic-creations.com/64-hair-conditioner-base
4 https://www.brambleberry.com/stephenson-organic-hair-condition-er-base-p6275.aspx

Hair Application Directions

After rinsing off your shampoo, apply the conditioner. Massage your hair and make sure that it's well-covered. Leave it on for three to five minutes. Rinse your hair with lukewarm water.

Storage of Product

Place the conditioner in a cool and dark place. You can also refrigerate it.

Shelf Life

This conditioner can last up to two months.

Recipe #27

Honey and Olive Oil Mix

Ingredient List

- 2 tablespoons of extra virgin oil
- 2 tablespoons of jojoba oil
- ½ cup of honey

Step-by-step Instructions

1. Combine the jojoba oil, extra virgin oil, and honey in a bowl.

2. Stir well.

3. Place the conditioner in a small dark glass bottle.

Hair Application Directions

After you shampoo, massage the conditioner on your hair. Apply a generous amount of this conditioner on the tip of your hair. Wait for five to ten minutes. Then, rinse off the conditioner using lukewarm water.

STORAGE OF PRODUCT
    Store the product in a dark and cool place.

SHELF LIFE
    This conditioner stays good for up to two weeks.

Recipe #28

Coconut Oil Instant Conditioner

INGREDIENT LIST
- 3 cups of coconut oil
- 5 drops of lavender essential oil

STEP-BY-STEP INSTRUCTIONS
1. Combine the coconut oil and the lavender oil in a small bowl.
2. Stir well.

HAIR APPLICATION DIRECTIONS
    After rinsing your shampoo, apply the conditioner on your hair. Massage your scalp and make sure that every part of your hair is covered. Leave the conditioner on for five minutes. Rinse off with cold water.

STORAGE OF PRODUCT
    Place the conditioner in a small dark bottle. Store in the refrigerator.

SHELF LIFE
    This condition can last up to one week.

Recipe #29

Cedarwood Moisturizing Conditioner

INGREDIENT LIST
- 1 cup of jojoba oil
- 3 drops of cedarwood oil
- 2 tablespoons of virgin coconut oil

STEP-BY-STEP INSTRUCTIONS
1. Combine all the ingredients in a bowl.
2. Stir well and then, store in a small dark glass bottle.

HAIR APPLICATION DIRECTIONS
After applying your shampoo, massage the conditioner into your hair – from roots to tips. Leave the conditioner on for three minutes. Then, rinse off using lukewarm water.

STORAGE OF PRODUCT
Keep the conditioner in a cool, dark place.

SHELF LIFE
This mixture normally lasts for up to two weeks. But, it could last longer when refrigerated.

Recipe #30

Clary Sage Anti-Balding and Moisturizing Conditioner

INGREDIENT LIST
- 5 tablespoons of coconut oil
- 10 drops of clary sage oil
- ½ cup of jojoba oil

STEP-BY-STEP INSTRUCTIONS
1. Mix the ingredients in a bowl.
2. Stir well.
3. Place in a small dark glass bottle.

HAIR APPLICATION DIRECTIONS
After rinsing off the shampoo, squeeze out the remaining water from your hair. Apply the conditioner from root to tip. Massage well. Be sure to leave the conditioner on for five to ten minutes. Rinse your hair using cold water.

STORAGE OF PRODUCT
Place the product in a dark and cool place. You can also refrigerate it to increase its shelf life.

SHELF LIFE
This can last up to two weeks. It can last up to a month when refrigerated.

Recipe #31

Lemon Instant Conditioner

INGREDIENT LIST
- 10 drops of lemon essential oil
- 1 cup of jojoba oil

STEP-BY-STEP INSTRUCTIONS
1. Place the jojoba oil in a small dark glass bottle.
2. Add ten drops of lemon essential oil.
3. Close the bottle and mix well.
4. Let the mixture sit for at least three hours before using.

HAIR APPLICATION DIRECTIONS
After applying shampoo, massage the conditioner onto your scalp. Leave it on for about ten minutes. Then, rinse your hair using lukewarm water.

STORAGE OF PRODUCT
Store the product in a dark and cool place. You can also refrigerate it.

SHELF LIFE
This conditioner can last up to three weeks. It will last up to two months when refrigerated.

Leave In Conditioner

Recipe #32

Coconut and Avocado Oil Conditioner

INGREDIENT LIST
- 1 cup of water
- 2 tablespoons of avocado oil
- 1 tablespoon of aloe vera gel
- 1 cup of coconut oil

STEP-BY-STEP INSTRUCTIONS
1. Place the water in a bowl.
2. Add the aloe vera gel, coconut oil, and avocado oil.
3. Mix well.
4. Pour the conditioner into a plastic container.

HAIR APPLICATION DIRECTIONS
Massage this conditioner into your hair. Then, blow dry your hair. Leave the conditioner on until the next wash.

STORAGE OF PRODUCT
Store this conditioner in the fridge.

SHELF LIFE
This conditioner can last up to two weeks.

Recipe #32

Jojoba Oil Leave-In Conditioner

INGREDIENT LIST
- 2 cups of aloe vera juice
- 2 tablespoons of jojoba oil
- 2 cups of coconut water

STEP-BY-STEP INSTRUCTIONS
1. Place the aloe vera juice in a bowl.
2. Add the coconut water and jojoba oil.
3. Mix well.
4. Transfer the conditioner into a plastic container.

HAIR APPLICATION DIRECTIONS
After washing your hair, apply the conditioner from root to tip. Leave it on until the next wash.

STORAGE OF PRODUCT
Store this leave in conditioner in the refrigerator.

SHELF LIFE
This conditioner lasts for up to two days.

Recipe #33

· ·
Lavender Leave-In Conditioner
· ·

INGREDIENT LIST
- 3 tablespoons of jojoba oil
- 3 tablespoons of shea butter
- ½ cup of coconut milk
- 5 drops of lavender oil

STEP-BY-STEP INSTRUCTIONS
1. Place the coconut oil in a plastic container.
2. Add the jojoba oil.
3. Add the shea butter and mix well.
4. Add the lavender oil.
5. Close the container.
6. Wait for an hour before using the conditioner.

HAIR APPLICATION DIRECTIONS
After washing your hair, apply a handful of this conditioner into your hair. Comb your hair afterwards. Leave it on until the next wash.

STORAGE OF PRODUCT
Refrigerate the conditioner to lengthen its shelf life.

SHELF LIFE
This leave-in conditioner can last up to two months.

Recipe #34

Tea Tree Oil Leave-In Conditioner

INGREDIENT LIST
- ½ cup of coconut milk
- 5 tablespoons of tea tree oil
- 3 tablespoons of aloe vera oil
- 1 cup of shea butter
- 2 tablespoons of jojoba oil
- 2 drops of ylang ylang oil

STEP-BY-STEP INSTRUCTIONS
1. Place the coconut oil in the bowl.
2. Add the shea butter and mix well.
3. Add the aloe vera oil, jojoba oil, and tea tree oil.
4. Mix well.
5. Place the conditioner in a dark glass bottle.

HAIR APPLICATION DIRECTIONS
After washing your hair, apply the conditioner on your hair. Comb your hair and leave the conditioner on until the next wash.

STORAGE OF PRODUCT
Store this conditioner in the refrigerator.

SHELF LIFE
This mixture can last up to three days.

Recipe #35

Rosemary and Avocado Leave-In Conditioner

INGREDIENT LIST
- 3 tablespoons of avocado oil
- 1 cup of shea butter
- 10 drops of rosemary essential oil

STEP-BY-STEP INSTRUCTIONS
1. Place the shea butter in a bowl.
2. Add the avocado oil.
3. Then, add the rosemary essential oil.
4. Mix well.
5. Store in a plastic or metal container.

HAIR APPLICATION DIRECTIONS
Apply the conditioner then massage and comb your hair. Leave the conditioner on for one day.

STORAGE OF PRODUCT
You can store it in a cool and dark place. But, you can also refrigerate it.

SHELF LIFE
This conditioner can last up to three weeks. It can even last up to a month if refrigerated.

Hair Conditioning Treatment

Summary and Recommendations

If you're still wondering which conditioners and recipes you should try, this table will help you out:

Conditioner	Benefits	Hair Types	Duration of Application	Frequency of Use
Rinse Out/ Instant Conditioner	Moisturizes the hair, making your hair more manageable and shiny.	Normal, Dry, or Oily Hair	3 to 5 minutes, but you can leave it on for up to 10 minutes	Once every three days or twice a week
Deep Conditioner	Moisturizes the hair, repairs damage, treats scalp issues	Damaged, treated, color-treated hair	30 minutes to one hour	Twice a month or as needed
Leave In Conditioner	Makes the hair more manageable	Frizzy and unmanageable hair	Leave on the hair until the next wash	Twice a week or as needed
Acid Rinse	It reduces dandruff and balances the pH levels of your hair.	Irritated and frizzy hair	10 to 40 minutes	Once a week
Beer Rinse	Moisturizes the hair and promotes hair growth. Makes your hair shiny.	Balding and dry hair	30 to 40 minutes	Twice or once a month
Herbal Rinse	Improves the overall health of your hair and promotes hair growth	Stressed and unhealthy hair	30 to 40 minutes	Once a week

Hair Condition	Hair Recipes to Try
Normal	Recipe #22, Recipe #23, Recipe #24, Recipe #25, Recipe #32, Recipe #33, Recipe #35
Dry	Recipe #4, Recipe #5, Recipe #7, Recipe #9, Recipe #26, Recipe #27, Recipe #29, Recipe #30, Recipe #34
Color-treated	Recipe #16
Damaged	Recipe #7, Recipe #8, Recipe #13, Recipe #26, Recipe #29, Recipe #34
Oily	Recipe #11, Recipe #12, Recipe #14, Recipe #18, Recipe #19, Recipe #28, Recipe #31
Breakage	Recipe #12, Recipe #17
Frizzy and Hard to Manage	Recipe #1, Recipe #5, Recipe #30
Tangled	Recipe #2
Weak	Recipe #3
Stressed	Recipe #8
Dandruff and Irritated Scalp	Recipe #6, Recipe #20, Recipe #34
Dull	Recipe #14, Recipe #27
Dark Hair	Recipe #15
Red Hair	Recipe #16
Thin or Balding Hair	Recipe #10, Recipe #15, Recipe #20, Recipe #21, Recipe #28, Recipe #30

Benefits of Ingredients Found in Recipes

The ingredients contained in this book are all natural. Of course, it's important that you learn about the ingredients and their benefits (especially when you're finally thinking of creating your own hair-revitalizing concoctions) – and that's why we came up with this quick guide:

Apple Cider Vinegar

Dandruff is often caused by external factors such as dry weather, using the wrong shampoo, using hot water when rinsing the hair, and washing the hair too frequently. Apple cider vinegar is a powerful hair rinse ingredient that prevents dandruff.

In addition, apple cider vinegar is a natural detangler. It reduces frizz and improves your hair's shine and gloss. It prevents hair breakage and split ends. So, it's perfect for brittle hair.

Aloe Vera

Aloe vera is packed with proteolytic enzymes, which give it the power to get rid of dead cells on the scalp. It helps prevent hair fall and dandruff. It even makes it easier to manage oily and frizzy hair.

Avocado

Avocado is one of the healthiest food items in the world. It is incredibly nutritious as it contains significant amounts of vitamin K, vitamin B5, vitamin B6, vitamin E, and potassium. In fact, the avocado contains more potassium than bananas.

Avocado oil can do wonders for your hair. It moisturizes and soothes your scalp. No wonder that it's a common hair conditioner ingredient. It promotes hair growth and prevents dandruff, too.

Baking Soda

You can find baking soda in many health and beauty products. This kitchen item controls the oil production in your scalp, making it perfect for people with oily hair.

Banana

Banana is rich in vitamins and minerals. It's a natural moisturizer and it is best for dry hair. It is rich in potassium and other minerals that naturally soften the hair, making it more manageable.

Beer

A lot of people say that beer isn't good for one's health. But, it contains a lot of vitamins and minerals that are actually good for you. Beer stimulates hair growth and increases the blood circulation in the scalp.

Black Tea

Black tea is rich in antioxidants. It contains caffeine, which helps decrease dihydrotesterone or DHT – a hormone that causes hair loss. Black tea increases the volume and thickness of hair. However, you should only apply black tea on your hair once a month. Applying black tea too often may prevent hair growth.

Burdock Root

Burdock root has been used for medicinal purposes in many cultures for centuries. It purifies hair and promotes hair growth. It contains various nutrients such as essential fatty acids, vitamin A, and mucilage that improves hair health.

Cayenne Pepper

Cayenne pepper improves blood circulation in your scalp. It's also loaded with components beneficial to hair, such as capsaicin, niacin, thiamine, folic acid, vitamin C, fatty oils, vitamin A, and phylloquinone. It even contains potassium which hydrates your scalp. This spicy herb moisturizes and strengthens hair, while keeping dandruff under control.

Chamomile Tea

Chamomile tea contains a cocktail of powerful antioxidants. It lightens your hair and helps prevent dandruff.

Cocoa Powder

Yes, you can use chocolate on your hair. Cocoa powder contains nutrients such as magnesium, protein, thiamine, and riboflavin that are good for your hair.

Coca-Cola

Coke is a powerful and cheap hair rinse that increases hair volume, giving you big and natural waves.

Coconut Milk

Coconut milk is a natural hair conditioner. It is packed with vitamins and minerals such as iron, vitamin E, vitamin B3, vitamin B5, phosphorous, and magnesium. It restores the shine of dry and damaged hair. It also treats irritated and itchy scalp. It's also known to strengthen brittle hair and minimize split ends.

Coconut oil

Coconut oil is rich in lauric acid that's also found in breast milk. This powerful compound prevents protein loss in the hair. It also penetrates hair quickly, meaning it provides immediate results.

Coconut oil helps control dandruff, but it may clog the pores in your scalp if you use it too often. For best results, combine coconut oil with other ingredients such as yogurt and honey.

Cedarwood Oil

This essential oil has a masculine and woody scent. Cedarwood oil increases blood circulation in the scalp. It makes your hair shine and it also promotes hair growth by stimulating your scalp.

Clary Sage Oil

Clary sage is a beautiful plant that bears pink and lilac flowers. It has a musky scent. It contains a chemical called phytoestrogen, which helps prevent balding. It also reduces oil production and helps control dandruff. Furthermore, this wonder oil helps control frizz, so it's ideal for curly and unmanageable hair.

Comfrey Root

Comfrey root moisturizes the hair and prevents hair loss. It is also a potent hair dye.

Eggs

Eggs contain fatty acids that moisturize the hair. It also helps manage frizzy hair. If you have dry hair, it's best to use egg yolks. But, if you have oily hair, you may want to use egg whites instead.

Extra Virgin Coconut Oil

This mainly improves the luster of hair. However, it also has anti-inflammatory properties that alleviates scalp irritation. It makes the hair effortlessly shiny and smooth.

Geranium Oil

Geranium oil is known to strengthen hair. Its relaxing scent is a bonus you'll surely appreciate.

Grapeseed Oil

Grapeseed oil is a natural hair conditioner. It reduces dermatitis and dandruff. It also contains powerful antioxidants that prevent the production of DHT – a hormone that causes hair loss. Aside from that, it promotes hair growth by relaxing the hair follicles.

This oil contains vitamin E that strengthens hair. So, if you have brittle hair, it's a good idea to use grapeseed oil as your hair conditioner.

Green Tea

Green tea strengthens hair. It also contains panthenol (vitamin B) – a common hair conditioner ingredient.

Furthermore, green tea is loaded with an antioxidant called EGCG, which stimulates hair growth and blocks a baldness-causing hormone called dihydrotestosterone (DHT).

Honey

Honey is a natural hair conditioner and it is a natural hair highlighter as it slowly releases hydrogen peroxide, making hair lighter. It prevents hair loss, too.

Horsetail

Horsetail promotes hair growth and strengthens hair.

Jojoba Oil

Jojoba oil prevents hair loss. It also helps you grow new hair by dissolving the clogs and debris that prevent your follicles from growing your hair.

Jojoba oil is a potent hair moisturizer and it helps control dandruff. It relieves scalp psoriasis by cleansing the scalp. It tames frizzy, dull, and dry hair. Massaging jojoba oil into your scalp improves blood circulation. It also helps preserve hair color.

Juniper Berry Oil

This essential oil has a sweet fruity scent that you can't simply get enough of. It blends well with other essential oils. It improves hair and scalp heath because of its strong antiseptic properties. It strengths brittle hair and prevents hair loss.

Lavender Oil

Lavender oil is sweet and it has a number of therapeutic benefits. It promotes hair growth and keeps hair from falling out. You can also mix it with different essential oils. Furthermore, it keeps hair shiny and it helps control dandruff.

Lemon

We all know that lemon is rich in vitamin C. It is acidic in nature but restores pH balance. It's good for your scalp. You can mix it with other ingredients such as henna, yogurt pack, aloe vera, extra virgin oil, egg, and coconut oil.

Lemon Grass Essential Oil

This essential oil has strong antifungal and antiviral properties. Lemon grass oil is perfect for those who are having scalp issues. It prevents dandruff by eliminating the dandruff-causing yeast.

Mayonnaise

Mayonnaise is a powerful hair moisturizer. It helps maintain the pH balance of your hair. It also helps prevent breakage and repairs damage.

Nettle

Nettle promotes hair growth so it is a perfect remedy for hair loss. Likewise, it helps treat scalp issues such as dandruff.

Olive Oil

Olive oil reduces dandruff and split ends. It also helps you manage your hair and reduce fly-aways. It contains antioxidants, vitamin E, and vitamin A that protect the keratin in the hair. It makes your hair softer and manageable.

Peppermint Oil and Leaves

This essential oil has an invigorating scent. It promotes hair growth and improves the thickness of your hair. It makes the hair follicles stronger so it's perfect for brittle hair. Keep in mind though, that you shouldn't apply this oil on young children.

You can also use peppermint leaves as a hair conditioner ingredient.

Rooibois Tea

This powerful tea is great for weight loss. But, it also has the power to preserve the color of the hair. It is great for women with light brown or red hair.

Raspberry Leaves

Raspberry leaves contain folic acid that promotes hair growth, making your hair shinier and healthier. They also contain vitamin C that improves scalp health.

Rose Essential Oil

Rose oil is a natural aphrodisiac and it is used in perfume production. It moisturizes your hair and prevents scalp dryness.

Rosehip Oil

Rosehip oil is best for thinning hair. In fact, many hair care experts call it the elixir for fine hair since it has a strengthening effect. It's also non-greasy so it's best for dry hair. This oil contains fatty acids that soothe scalp problems, while increasing hair luster and elasticity.

Rosemary Essential Oil

Rosemary is a natural preservative. If you want your homemade conditioner to last longer, it's a good idea to add rosemary oil. This amazing essential oil also prevents premature baldness.

Sandalwood Oil

This essential oil has a musky scent and helps reduce split ends. It also makes hair smoother and more manageable.

Shea butter

Shea butter is one of the most common ingredients in organic hair and skin care products. It contains fatty acids that naturally moisturize hair.

Strawberry

Strawberries moisturize your hair, making your hair shinier and silkier. It also contains manganese, copper, and magnesium that eliminates the fungus in your scalp.

Sweet Almond Oil

This oil is great for dandruff treatment. It contains large amounts of vitamin A and E that are both good for hair. It contains fatty acids that moisturize hair from the inside. It makes your hair shiny, bright, and silky looking.

Tea Tree Oil

Tea tree oil cleanses the hair and scalp. It promotes hair growth so it's good for those who have thin hair. This essential oil also fights dandruff.

Thyme

Thyme has a strong anti-fungal and anti-bacterial properties that help control dandruff. It is rich in potassium, calcium, manganese, selenium, and iron that improve hair health.

Vanilla Essential Oil

Vanilla has a sweet scent that you can't get enough of. It helps you achieve smooth, shiny, and silky hair. It blends well with jojoba and castor oil.

Vegetable Glycerin

You can find vegetable glycerin in many skincare products. But, it is also good for your hair. Vegetable glycerin is a natural moisturizer that blends well with many essential oils. It retains the moisture of the hair and stops dandruff.

Virgin Coconut Oil

Virgin coconut oil contains nutrients, vitamins, and fatty acids such as saturated fatty acids, lauric acid, capric acid, oleic acid, vitamin K, and vitamin E.

Witch Hazel

Witch hazel rejuvenates hair, restoring its luster. It stabilizes the oil in your scalp without drying your hair. It treats dandruff and improves blood circulation in the scalp.

Ylang ylang Oil

What's amazing about the ylang ylang oil is that it stimulates hair growth. So, if you want to make your hair longer in a short period of time, this is an excellent choice.

Yogurt

Yogurt promotes hair growth, helps control dandruff and frizz, and balances the scalp's pH level.

Conclusion

I hope that the recipes contained in this book have helped you deal with your hair issues. Rest assured that these recipes were carefully chosen to help you achieve shinier, healthier, and more beautiful hair.

Here are a few final reminders before you try out the recipes in this book:

* Examine your hair thoroughly and determine if it's oily, dry, or damaged. That way, you'll be able to pick the right hair care recipes to try.
* If you have oily hair, avoid massaging the carrier oils on your scalp for longer than 30 seconds.
* If you plan to make a lot of conditioners at home, invest in high quality containers. You'll find those at your local beauty stores. You can purchase them online.
* See how your hair responds to these homemade conditioners. If your scalp feels itchy after applying a homemade conditioner, see your dermatologist right away.

Thank you and good luck!

Resources

* http://www.motherearthliving.com/Health-and-Wellness/body-and-soul-herbal-hair-rinses

* http://www.easy-aromatherapy-recipes.com/natural-hair-conditioner.html

* http://www.top10homeremedies.com/kitchen-ingredients/10-natural-ingredients-for-healthy-hair-skin-nails.html

* http://curlsunderstood.com/benefits-of-honey-for-natural-hair/

* http://www.stylishwalks.com/incredible-benefits-strawberries-hair-health-skin/

* https://www.organicfacts.net/health-benefits/essential-oils/vanilla-essential-oil.html

* http://food.ndtv.com/beauty/10-amazing-coconut-milk-benefits-for-hair-face-and-skin-1421580

* http://www.naturallivingideas.com/coconut-oil-for-hair/

* http://www.hairbuddha.net/scalp-elixir-for-fine-thinning-hair/

* http://www.livestrong.com/article/277391-lemon-juice-for-a-hair-rinse/

* http://www.seventeen.com/beauty/hair/a30377/coca-cola-hair-wash/

* https://www.babble.com/beauty/10-ways-to-use-apple-cider-vinegar-for-hair/

* http://www.rivertea.com/blog/5-ways-tea-benefits-hair/

* http://www.goodhealthacademy.com/health-benefits/jojoba-oil-for-hair/

* http://www.stylecraze.com/articles/health-benefits-of-chamomile-tea/#gref

* http://stylecaster.com/beauty/hair-rinses/#slide-7

* https://www.organicfacts.net/health-benefits/beverage/chamomile-tea-benefits-uses.html

* http://www.naturallivingideas.com/coconut-oil-for-hair/

* http://www.humblebeeandme.com/faqs/whats-the-difference-between-a-vinegaracidic-rinse-and-conditioner/

* https://www.curejoy.com/content/benefits-of-olive-oil-for-health-skin-and-hair/

www.ingramcontent.com/pod-product-compliance
Lightning Source LLC
Chambersburg PA
CBHW060756260726
48660CB00002B/651